TENKIDOKAN

Stages of Qi Cultivation

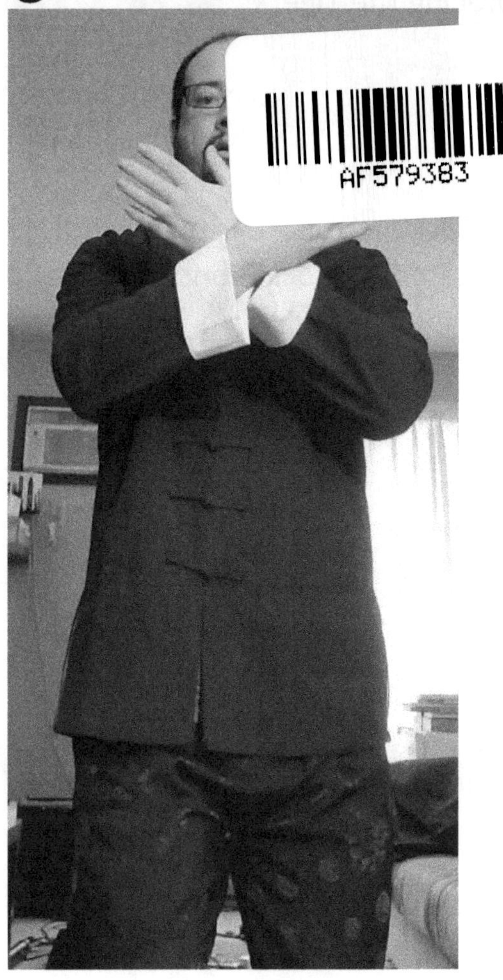

Wu Ming

The front cover photo is the author embracing the Tiger.

The above Photo is the Author Embracing the Tiger.

The back cover photo is the Author doing Golden Rooter/Cock Stands on One Leg.

TENKIDOKAN

Stages of Qi Cultivation

BY

Wu Ming

PUBLISHED BY

BONG-BONG

TENKIDOKAN

Distributed globally by Amazon.

1 2 3 4 5 6 7 8 9 10

Ming, Wu
Stages of Qi Cultivation

This text is for advice only. Seek the direction of a qualified teacher for training.

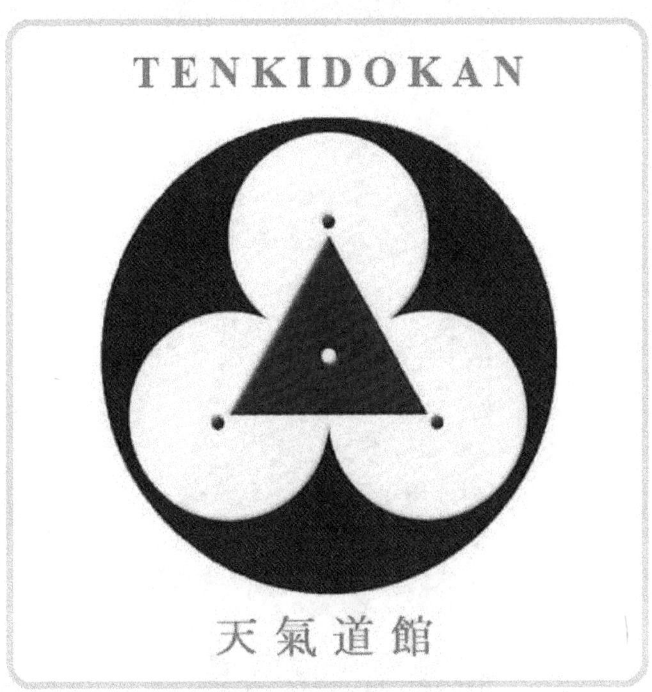

About the Author

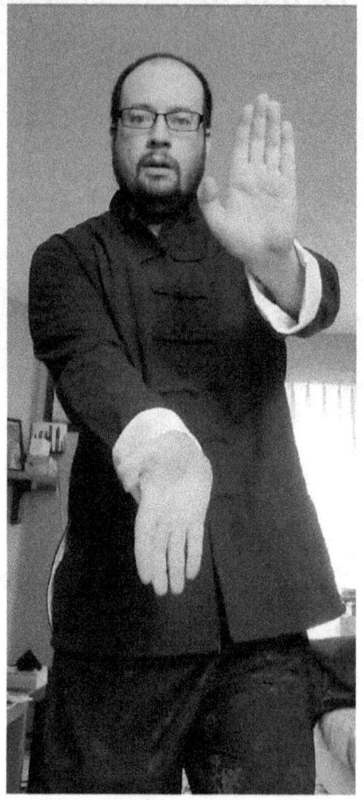

Wu Ming is more than a Qi Gong student and teacher. He studied Anthropology, Philosophy, Asian Studies, and Classical History at the University of Manitoba in Manitoba Canada.

He has been studying Qi Gong and Martial Arts since 2013 and is a certified Qi Gong and

Tai Ji Qi Gong instructor with the Tenkidokan School of Energy Arts.

His mission in life is to spread the ancient wisdom of Asia to the West and to demystify to Energy Arts by presenting Qi Gong in practical terms that are much more suited for a Western audience.

Wu Ming also sees great value in showing how science and the ancient Energy Arts like Qi Gong both work on the same principles. It is one of his missions in life to show that the Energy Arts obey the physical laws of the Universe and that the ancient mystical explanations were the best explanations the ancients could come up with using the tools available to them.

DEDICATION

This text is dedicated to all students of the Energy Arts and Qi Gong.

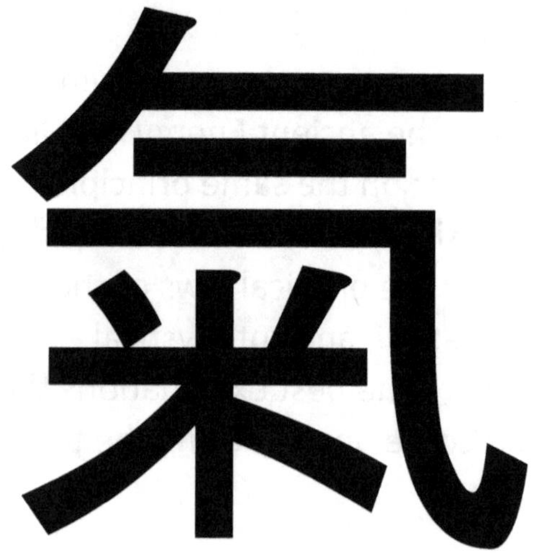

Table of Contents

Introduction

Qi is energy. It is any energy. It is common to see Qi as life force energy, spiritual energy, or magical energy. Two of these terms are correct. The third term has no evidence beyond trickery and illusion.

Qi is any form of energy. Since Qi is any form of energy and a living organism needs energy to be alive, then Qi being life force is an ok description. From the smallest single celled organism to the largest organism, the one thing they all require to be alive is energy. Life energy is a mix of different types of energies and thus Qi as life force is a mix of all these energies. As my Qi Gong Sifu Kevin Dewayne Hughes told me, "Qi is a catch all term for all the forms of energy and fluid flows in the body."

We all have a spiritual existence. No matter if you are an atheist or theist, we all have a spiritual component. The spirit may be the consciousness within our brain that dies when our brain dies. It may be a part of our existence beyond the physical body that never dies. No matter what view you take, the spirit needs energy to function. Therefore, Qi energy as spiritual energy is an ok description too.

Each person has his or her own personal Qi and then there is the Universal Qi. Even objects and phenomena within the Universe have Qi. Qi is everywhere and within everything.

In this text we will explore Qi development as taught to me by my Qi Gong Sifu Kevin Dewayne Hughes and his Tenkidokan School of Energy Arts.

Five Stages of Qi Development

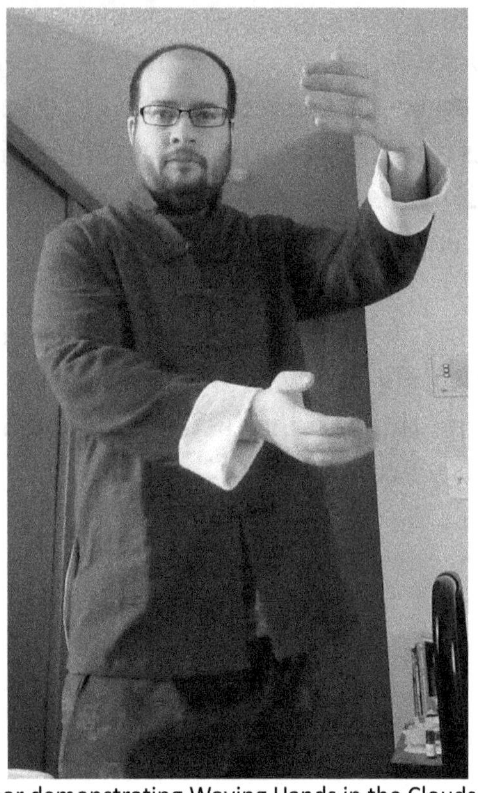

The Author demonstrating Waving Hands in the Clouds from Tai Ji Qi Gong

It does not matter if a person has never trained in or studied Qi Gong, which is a method of exercising and developing a person's internal energy system. The Qi will flow regardless. It does not matter if the person believes in Qi or not. The Qi will flow regardless.

The purpose of Qi Gong is to bring awareness of Qi so that a person can improve their Qi flow, Qi conversion, and Qi storage. As the student grows, the student studying Qi Gong will go through five stages of development.

First Stage – Gross External Shape

The first stage of development is the gross external shape. This is doing the postures and movements in a manor that looks correct. The postures may be off a little and the movements off a little. Despite any offness of the movements and postures, the layperson will see the person's form as matching the model form.

Second Stage – Fine External Shape

The second stage of development is the fine external shape. This is when the performer looks graceful in their movements. All the fine details of a posture or movement are present and near perfect.

Gracefulness in movement is an external testament to the internal energy flow. If the Qi flow is smooth then the movement will be graceful. If the Qi flow is chaotic, then the movement will also be chaotic. The way a person moves tells us how the energy is flowing in the person. Gracefulness in movement is one means that an instructor can gage a student's energy flow. Stiffness is another means an instructor can find places that the student has retarded energy flow.

Stage two also covers proper body alignment. The alignment of the spine and other joints in the body physically control the body's energy gates. Too little range of motion and the energy gates are too closed. Too much range of motion and the energy gates are too open. The body's energy system needs the energy gates open just right. My Qi Gong Sifu Kevin Dewayne Hughes says to find the Goldilocks Zone for your energy gates and energy valves.

Flexibility of the skeletal muscles is another stage two development area. The energy flows better through flexible muscle tissues than it does through tense muscle tissue. This relates back to Yin and Yang. Make sure Yin and Yang are balanced. Find its Goldilocks Zone and target the middle.

Sifu Kevin Dewayne Hughes gives good discussion on the topic in his book:

Introduction to the Theory of Yin-Yang

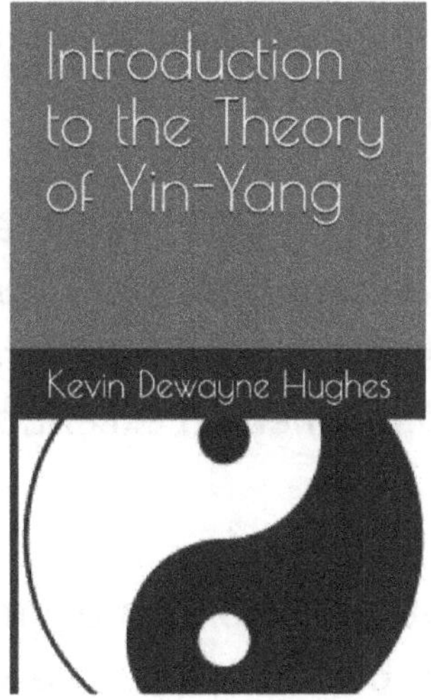

To the common observer, the person with good stage two will appear to them as a master. Yet this person is only two fifths of the way to mastery.

"A Warrior is more than just disciplined in fighting arts," Kevin Dewayne Hughes

Third Stage – Gross Internal Shape

The third stage of development is the gross internal shape. The gross internal shape involves the breath being coordinated with the movements. The speed of the breath controls the speed of the movement. The breath is out on closing, pushing, contracting, and sinking movements. The breath is in on opening, pulling, expanding, and rising movements.

There are exceptions to the above rules when it comes to the breath work. Your sifu will explain when these exceptions occur and help you understand when an exception should be made.

If you run out breath on a movement, just start the next breath cycle. Pause the form at the end of the movement and reset your breath by bringing the breath to the point of the finished movement. If the movement was an exhale movement, then get to the end of the exhale on the breath cycle and then resume the form with the inhale and start the next inhale movement. If the movement was an inhale movement, then get to the inhale on the breath cycle and then resume the form with the exhale and start the next exhale movement.

The breath is the external expression of the internal energy cycle.

Stage three is also characterized by postural alignments. These are external expressions that translate to enhanced energy flow. The enhancement of energy flow is due to the resulting relaxation.

Alignment 1
Open the chest. Opening the chest reduces restriction on the conception meridian. Pulling the shoulders back is one way to open the chest, but this action closes the back and retards the flow of energy along the governing meridian.

Alignment 2
Open the back. Opening the back reduces restriction on the governing meridian. Scrunching the shoulders forward is one way to open the back, but this action closes the

chest and retards the flow of energy along the conception meridian.

It seems that opening the one closes the other. The solution is to expand your thoracic cavity like a sliding door. When you inhale, instead of expanding the chest to the front, focus on opening the chest to the sides. This will open the chest and back at the same time. Now focus on the side way expansion to keep both the chest and back open while inhaling and exhaling. This is how you achieve alignment one and two together.

Alignment 3
Suspend the shoulders from the trunk. Let the tension melt out of the shoulders. Stop fighting gravity and let gravity lengthen the connective tissues in the shoulders.

Suspension of the shoulders cannot occur if the arms are plastered to the side of the body. Allow the arms to be away from the body ever so slightly. Keeping the arms plastered to the torso impedes the lengthening work of gravity. Therefore, imagine having an egg in your armpits. The egg should not be in any danger of being crushed. This will help to keep the arms off the torso just enough.

If the arms are too far away from the body, then muscular tension will engage as the muscles, rather than the skeletal structure, will need to work to support the weight of the arms. The egg can help here too. Have it so that the egg will not drop from the armpits. If the arms are such that the egg is barely held by the armpits, then the arm is in the best position to maximize relaxation in the shoulders. Maximized relaxation will result in maximized Qi flow through the shoulders.

Alignment 4

Sink the elbows. The elbows tend to flare out a little. This flaring to the sides, front, or back requires the shoulder muscles to work instead of relax. By sinking the elbow, the elbow will hang to the lowest point and reduce the stress on the shoulders.

Alignment 5

Suspend the head. The neck muscles work long and hard at keeping our heads upright and in place all day long. The constant tension in the neck impedes the flow of Qi.

Imagine that the top of the head is attached to a cable. From this connection point, imagine that the whole body hangs from there. The cervical vertebrae decompress and the neck muscles relax. The muscles go to a minimum energy usage point. Less energy being used by the muscles means more Qi can flow.

Muscular tension results in the storage of Qi instead of the flow of Qi. Tension needs more energy than relaxation and thus more energy stores into the muscles instead of flowing along the energy channel. Complete relaxation reduces the muscular energy use and thus more energy is allowed to pass by on the energy channel.

Alignment 6

Round the buttock. We stand a lot and it's the legs that support the whole body. The legs and buttock work hard and become stiff.

Rounding the buttocks helps to release the tension between the body and the legs.

Take a moment and focus on your buttock while standing. You will notice a lot of tension there. This tension results from the work the buttock does to keep you standing up.

Now relax the buttock and notice how it rounds out taking pressure off the energy gates to the legs and off the lower portion of the governing meridian.

There are other postural alignments and other points that go into this stage of Qi development. For now, use these to start your exploration of energy cultivation.

Please understand that relaxation, and not limpness, is the key to enhanced energy flow.

In general, the gross internal shape has physical twins to the energy that an observer can detect. Stage four has no physical twins.

Stage three, four, and five can be developed together. However, it is easier to develop stage five if stage four is already strong. It is also easier to develop stage four if stage three is already strong.

Stage two needs stage one developed first. If the gross external shape is missing, it is impossible to develop the fine external shape. A strong stage two will help stage three to get stronger faster even though stage three can start development with stage one.

Stage Four – Fine Internal Shape
Stage four of development is the fine internal stage. Visualizations are key to this stage. The first visualization is the microcosmic orbit. This is visualizing the flow of energy along the spine and the front side of the body.

The mind always leads the Qi. Wherever the mind visualizes the Qi that is where the Qi will concentrate in flow. This is one reason for looking at the hands during practice. Looking at the hand concentrates the mind on the hands so that it becomes easier for the mind to lead the Qi to the hands.

Even more energy can flow with the proper visualizations. When pushing and pulling, visualize a heavy box being pushed and pulled. This can cause the mind to send extra energy into the movement.

One way to understand this can be observed with dreams. If a person dreams of running, their heart races as if they were really running. The mind believes the body was actually running so the mind led the energy into the heart to beat faster.

There is a key component to stage four. The mind must believe the visualization is really happening. If the mind does not believe the visualization, then the mind will not lead extra Qi.

Emotions also impact the flow of Qi. This is why one should smile on the inside. A positive emotional state leads to better energy flow than a negative emotional state.

The flip side is martial Qi Gong. In martial Qi Gong, one wants to project destructive emotional intent into the techniques. The mind is capable of multiple simultaneous emotional states. Keep the main emotional state positive with the inward smile while projecting the negative emotional energy into the techniques.

Stage Five – Projection and Extension
Stage five is projection and extension of the Qi. It is not related to using the Force like a Jedi Knight. It is quite different as we will see.

Projection of the Qi means to extend it past the physical limits of the body. This is best accomplished with visualizations of the energy going beyond the physical body. When extending a reach, visualize the limb reaching beyond where it can physically reach. This is one of the secrets to the unbendable arm.

In martial Qi Gong, extend the energy of a technique beyond the surface and into the target. Sifu Kevin Dewayne Hughes is also a

Sensei of Okinawan Karate. He says that Karate has an internal energy aspect like the martial arts of Tai Chi, Hsing-I, and Ba Gua. He says that old Okinawan Karate projects negative and destructive emotional intent into techniques. He further says Okinawan Karate techniques do not target the surface presented. Instead, old Okinawan Karate targets the backside by going through the front side. That is, when hitting the solar plexus, the target is actually the backside of the spine. The backside of the spine is struck by entering at the solar plexus and going through the body to the other side. This does not mean that the fist will physically go through the body. What it means is that the intensity of the blow will cause deeper damage to the target than surfacing hitting will do.

Extension means to keep the Qi flowing. This can be seen with a novice runner. While they are running, the Qi is extending. As soon as they cross the finish line, they stop extending Qi. This results in them collapsing after crossing the finish line.

The experienced runner crosses the finish line and keeps extending Qi. They do not collapse but allow the body to slowly return to a rest state because they kept the Qi extending.

Stages of Qi Development Between the Hands

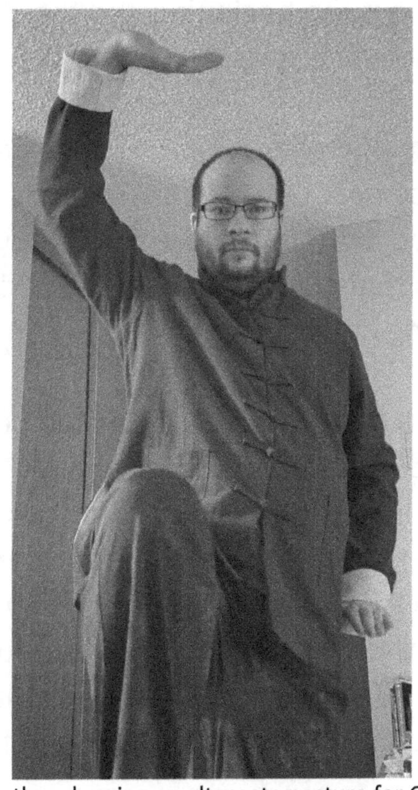

The Author showing an alternate posture for Golden Rooster/Cock Stands On One Leg

In the Tai Ji Qi Gong taught at the Tenkidokan, the first routine taught is called Qi Ball. The purpose of this form is to open the Qi gates, valves, and channels so that maximal projection and extension can occur. At the end, the strength of the Qi field in the hands is checked.

Stage zero is the beginning and the student will likely feel nothing out of the ordinary.

Stage one of development and the person will notice heat between their hands. It will not be too alarming to them and they may not even register that they are experiencing something out of the ordinary.

Stage two of development and the person will notice what feels like magnetic propulsion between their hands. Just like how a person can feel an invisible bubble between two magnets when the two north poles or the two south poles are brought together. The person will feel a similar magnetic bubble like force between their hands.

Stage three of development is essentially like stage two. In stage two the hands are required to be close together to feel the magnetic bubble. In stage three, the hands can be far apart and still feel the magnetic bubble.

Sifu Hughes says he got the magnetic bubble on his first go at Qi Ball when he learned it from his first Tai Ji teacher Sergio Ojeta. Seigung Ojeta did not tell Sifu Hughes what to experience. Sifu Hughes did not know what was going on when he felt the magnetic bubble.

Now one reason Sifu Hughes felt it on day one was because he had over a decade of Kikou under his belt. Kihou is Japanese Qi Gong and it is a part of old Okinawan Karate training. In Kikou they did not do exercises to check the Ki (Qi) strength like the Tai Ji was doing.

At first, Sifu Hughes looked for all sorts of explanations for what he was feeling. At first, he thought that since the hands were in close proximity and his Sifu, Sergio Ojeta, had him close his eyes for the exercise, that perhaps the brain knew the hands were close to touching but not touching and the brain interpreted that as the magnetic bubble.

As time went on, Sifu Hughes eventually got to stage three and he could feel the magnetic bubble between his hands at a distance beyond what would be feasible for a misinterpretation by the brain due to the close proximity of the hands to each other. It was at this point that Sifu Hughes started to realize that there was more to Qi than just some mystical explanation.

Stage four of development and the person will notice their hands tingle. Sifu Hughes hypothesizes that the brain interprets the extra energy at the nerve endings as the tingling sensation.

Stage five of development and the person will think that their hands are bigger and heavier than they really are. Sifu Hughes hypothesizes that the brain interprets all that extra energy as the hands being more massive, that is bigger and heavier than reality. His reasoning is that bigger hands will naturally have more energy in them. After all, matter is just congealed energy.

Sifu Hughes knows when someone hits stage two. He will have students checking their Qi at the end of Qi ball. When a student feels it for the first time, they will start looking around the room, then look back at their hands in bewilderment, then they look around the room again, then back to their hands...

Now Sifu Hughes does not tell the students what they might feel. He lets them self discover. He figures that a student discovering it is a more powerful teaching tool and removes psychological conditioning from the equation.

Some General Remarks About Qi Gong

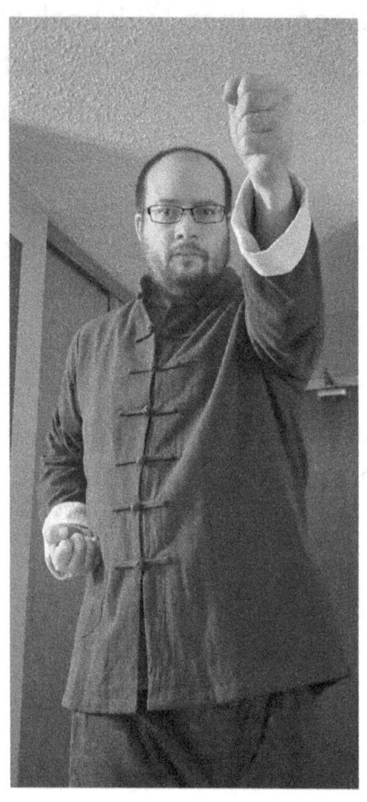

This shows a punch seen in Tai Ji Qi Gong. Tai Ji Qi Gong is derived from Tai Ji Quan Fa. Tai Ji Quan Fa is a Martial Art with a Military origin. Many movements in Tai Ji Qi Gong have combative applications just waiting to be explored. However, as Sifu Kevin Dewayne Hughes emphasizes, Martial Arts forms are a mixture of combative applications and health maintenance.

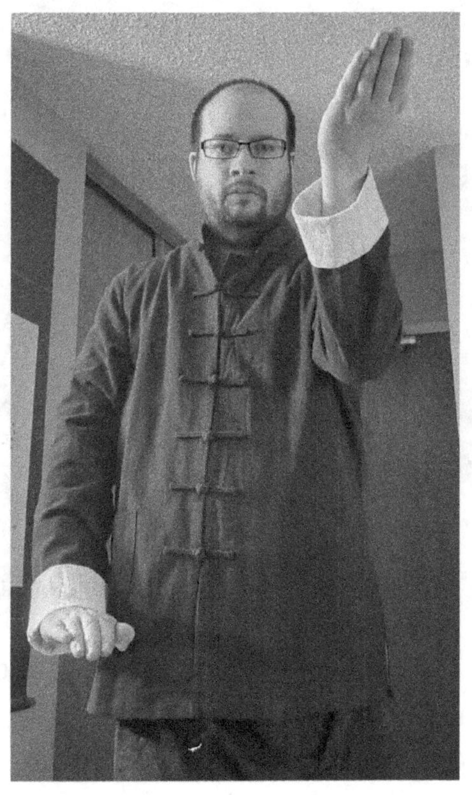

The alignments of each joint in a posture are critical to the flow of Qi. By placing the joints into the proper alignments, the associated energy gate will be opened to the optimal setting.

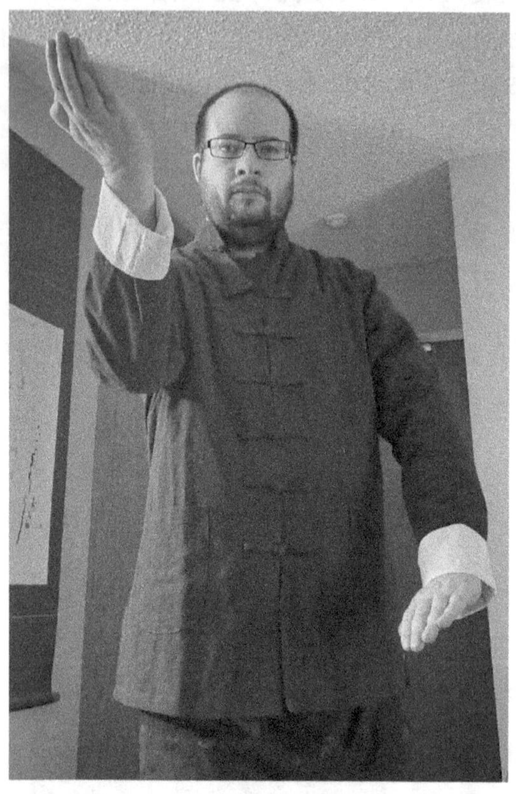

Notice this picture and the previous picture are similar. Despite the joints needing proper alignment, there can still be variation between schools as to how that alignment can be done. Remember that one school's or one teacher's way is not the only path to the top of the mountain.

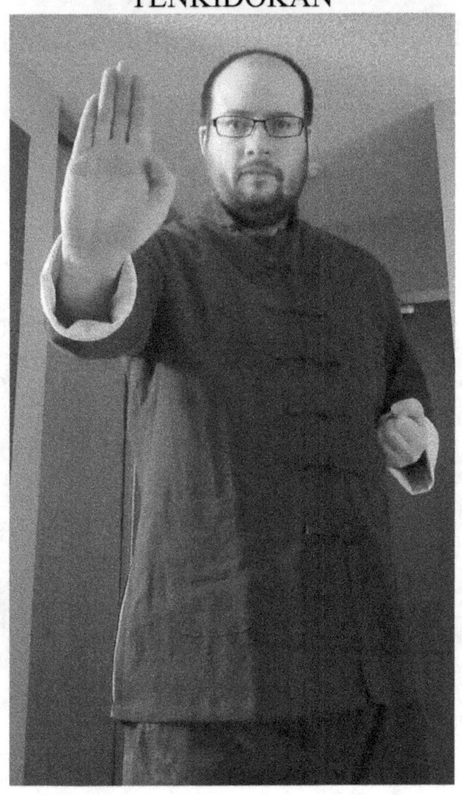

All forms practice in martial arts from Kung Fu to Karate have the goal of being Qi Gong routines and not just an imaginary fight against multiple opponents. In fact it is not an imaginary fight at all. As Sifu Hughes puts it, the forms are a catalog of combative techniques mixed in with movements that move the body through un-necessary ranges of motion for the purpose of maintaining and improving health.

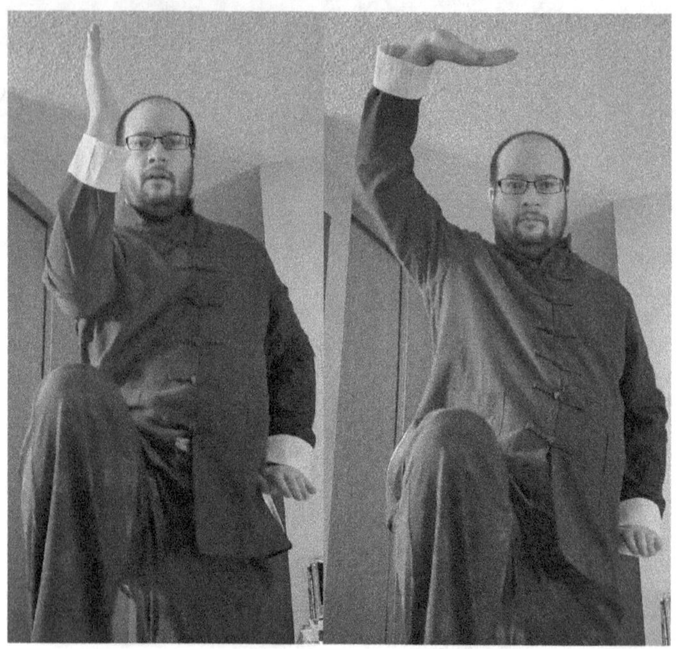

Take note that postures from different styles can be different. Both of these are Golden Rooster Stands on One Leg. They are simple style specific variations of that same pose.

It can also be that the exact same name for a posture or movement can have extremely different uses and functions to the point that the two are not related at all. Conversely, the same movement with the exact same use and function between two styles can have very different names.

Please keep this in mind with your training and explorations of an art or discipline in both the Energy Arts and the Martial Arts.

The Tenkidokan School of Energy Arts

The Tenkidokan is a school equivalent to a university founded by Kevin Dewayne Hughes. It has schools of Martial Arts, Energy Arts, Health & Fitness, Theology & Spirituality, and Science. It also has research arms for Martial Arts called the Koryu Bugei Hozon Kenkyukai and for Energy Arts called the Universal Energy Arts Society.

The Tenkidokan School of Martial Arts is the most famous division of the Tenkidokan. The Tenkidokan School of Energy Arts is the second most popular school.

The Universal Energy Arts Society works to unify the different ideologies of the various Energy Arts such as Qi Gong, Kikou, Reiki, Yoga and many more. The organization looks for what is similar and what is different. It then looks to find modern scientific explanations for the old ideas that are similar. The ideas that are different are explored to find out how to reconcile the difference or to discard the least likely versions of the different ideas. The ideas that cannot be explained with modern scientific understanding are tabled or discarded. In other word the goal of the Universal Energy Arts Society is to demystify the ancient Energy Arts.

For example, the concept of no touch knockouts was one area the Universal Energy Arts Society discarded and left it as a psychological manipulation by the no touch knockout masters. Sifu Kevin Dewayne Hughes said the concept was so laughable that he didn't even bother to test this one or table it. It immediately went into the trash bin.

The Universal Energy Arts Society is the research arm of the Tenkidokan School of Energy Arts. At this school, the arts of Qi Gong, Yoga, Meditation, Massage, and other Energy Arts are taught with both theory and skills. Students can become certified to teach these disciplines through the Tenkidokan School of Energy Arts.

Since the Tenkidokan is like a University, the founder Kevin Dewayne Hughes is not the only subject teacher. There are other teachers that teach subjects that the founder does not teach. There are also teachers that teach the same subjects as the founder. For example: both I and Sifu Hughes teach Qi Gong and Tai Ji Qi Gong for the Tenkidokan School of Energy Arts.

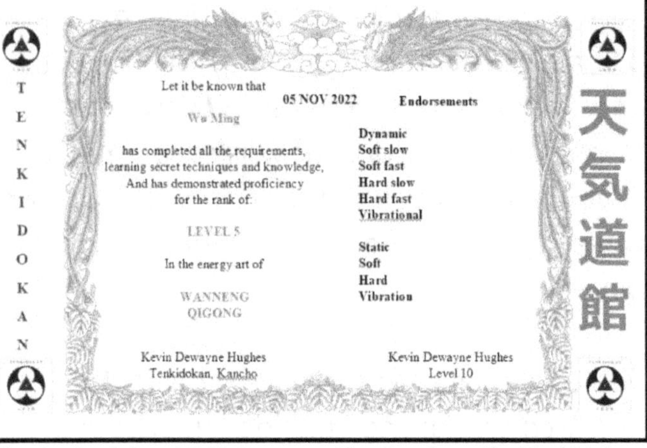

The Author's level 5 Qi Gong certification from the Tenkidokan School of Energy Arts

TENKIDOKAN

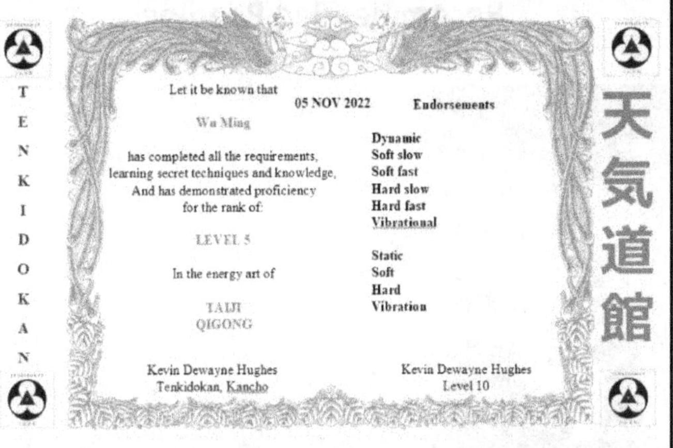

T E N K I D O K A N

天気道館

Let it be known that

05 NOV 2022

Wu Ming

has completed all the requirements,
learning secret techniques and knowledge,
And has demonstrated proficiency
for the rank of:

LEVEL 5

In the energy art of

TAIJI
QIGONG

Endorsements

Dynamic
Soft slow
Soft fast
Hard slow
Hard fast
Vibrational

Static
Soft
Hard
Vibration

Kevin Dewayne Hughes
Tenkidokan, Kancho

Kevin Dewayne Hughes
Level 10

The Author's Level 5 Tai Ji Qi Gong certification from the Tenkidokan School of Energy Arts

Recommended Reading

Books by my Sensei

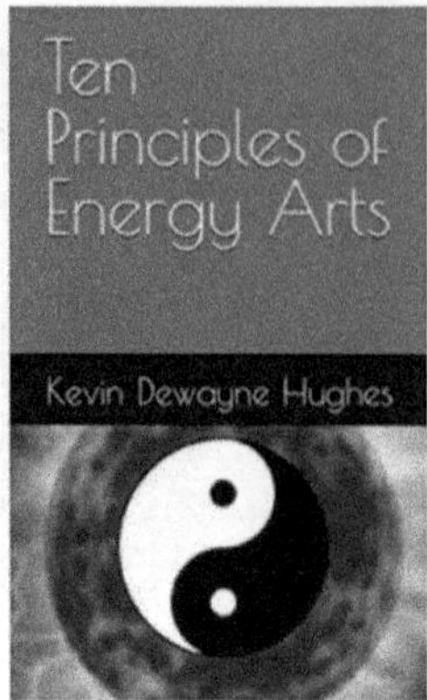

Ten Principles of Energy Arts
By: Kevin Dewayne Hughes
ISBN: 978-1696804592

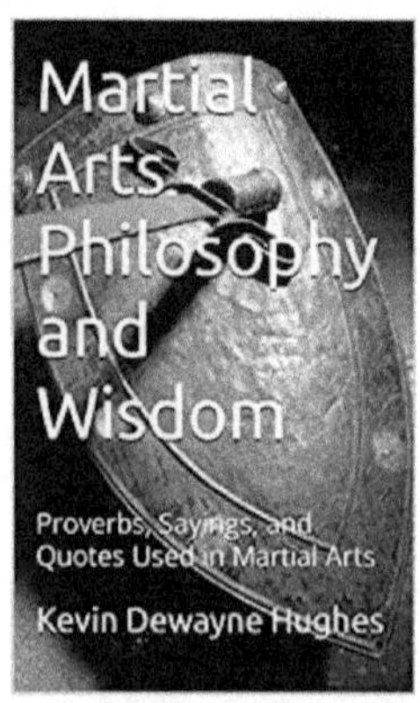

Martial Arts Philosophy and Wisdom: Proverbs, Sayings, and Quotes used in Martial Arts
By: Kevin Dewayne Hughes
ISBN: 979-8372057586

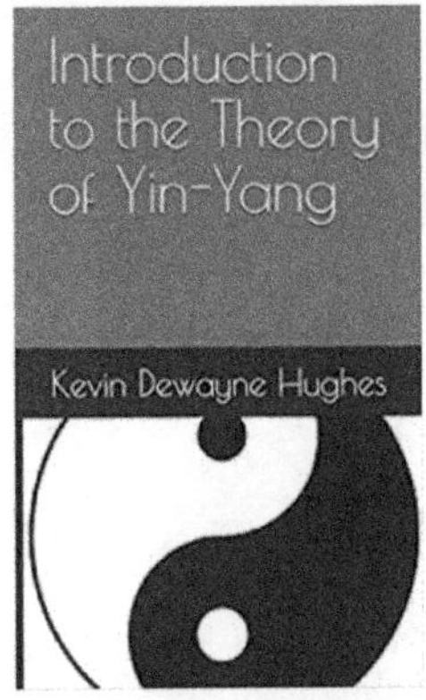

Introduction to the Theory of Yin-Yang
By: Kevin Dewayne Hughes
ISBN: 979-8667867869

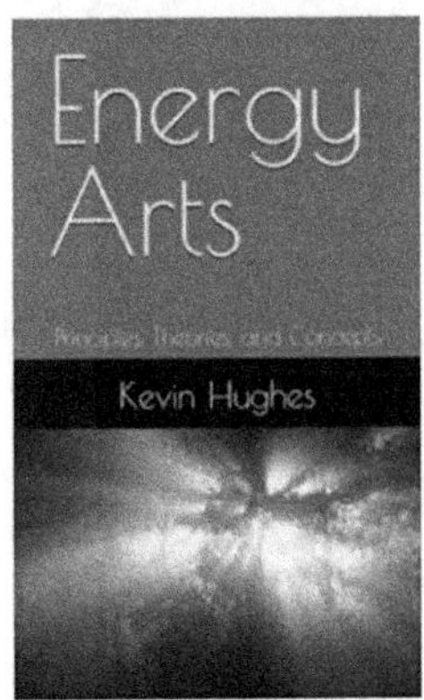

Energy Arts: Principles, Theories, and Concepts
By: Kevin Dewayne Hughes
ISBN: 979-8372102484

TENKIDOKAN

Books from

Bong Bong

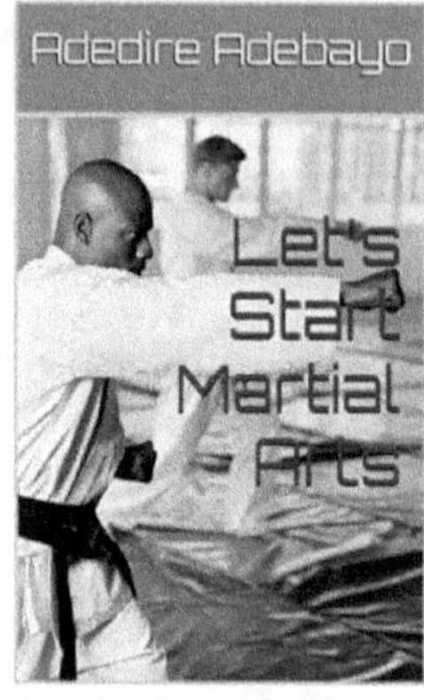

Let's Start Martial Arts

By: Adedire Sodiq Adebayo

ISBN: 979-8371257369

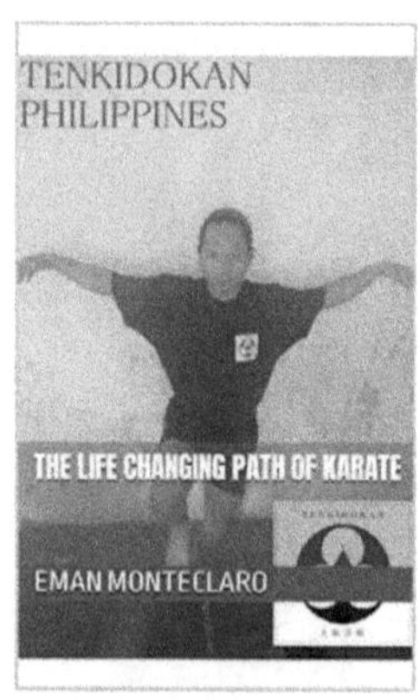

The Life Changing Path of Karate

By: Eman Monteclaro

ASIN: B0BRNYQ2DX

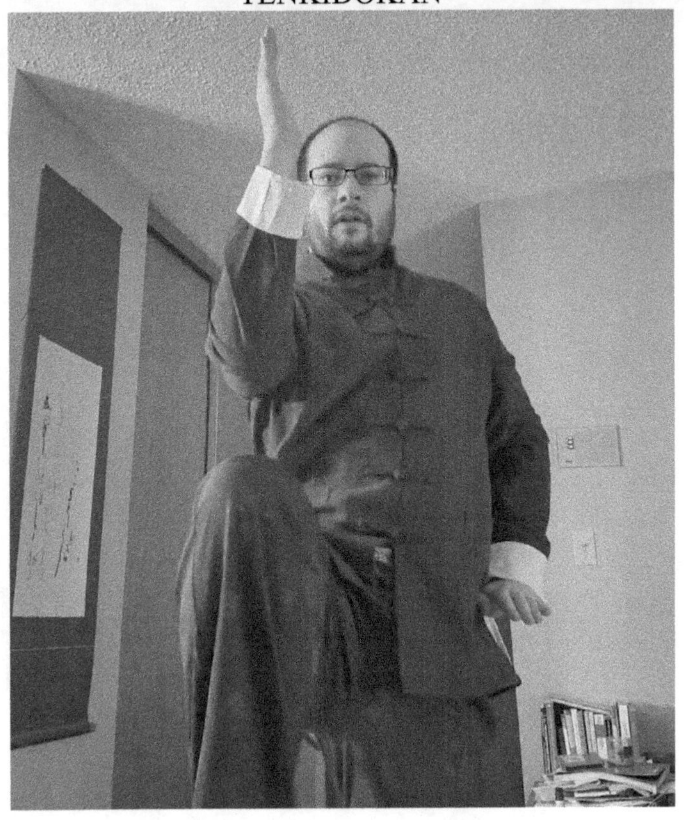

Back Cover Photo

www.ingramcontent.com/pod-product-compliance
Lightning Source LLC
LaVergne TN
LVHW020527160826
845677LV00015B/3941